This book is dedicated to a hero
I know – my nephew Parker.
I love you Buddy.

-*Aunt Mandy*

Our bodies are made up of trillions of teeny-tiny things called cells.

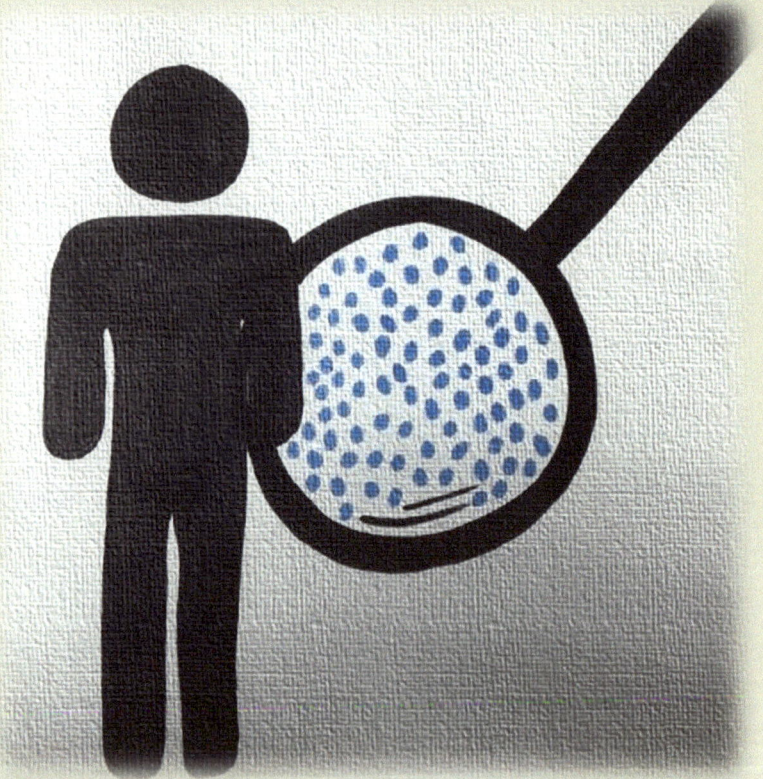

Many people call cells the "building blocks of life" because every single living thing is made of them.

Each cell in our body has it's very own job to do — just like your mom or dad.

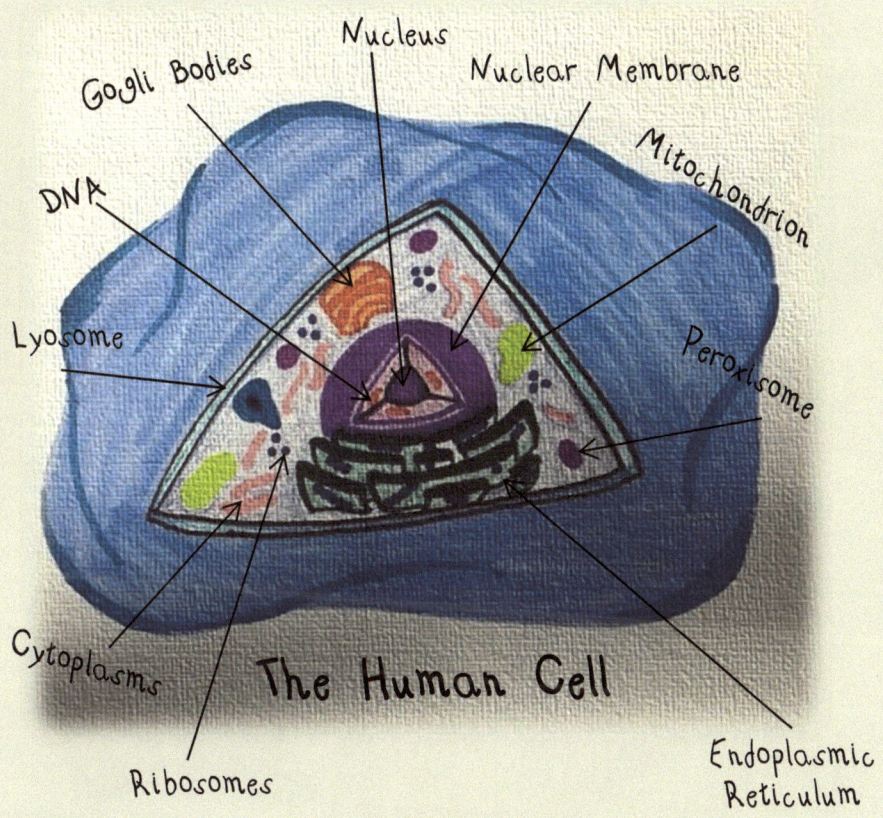

The Human Cell

Labels: Gogli Bodies, Nucleus, Nuclear Membrane, Mitochondrion, DNA, Lyosome, Peroxisome, Cytoplasms, Ribosomes, Endoplasmic Reticulum

When your parents go to work, they have a boss who tells them what to do.

Cells also have a boss, but it is not a person. Cells are told what to do by DNA.

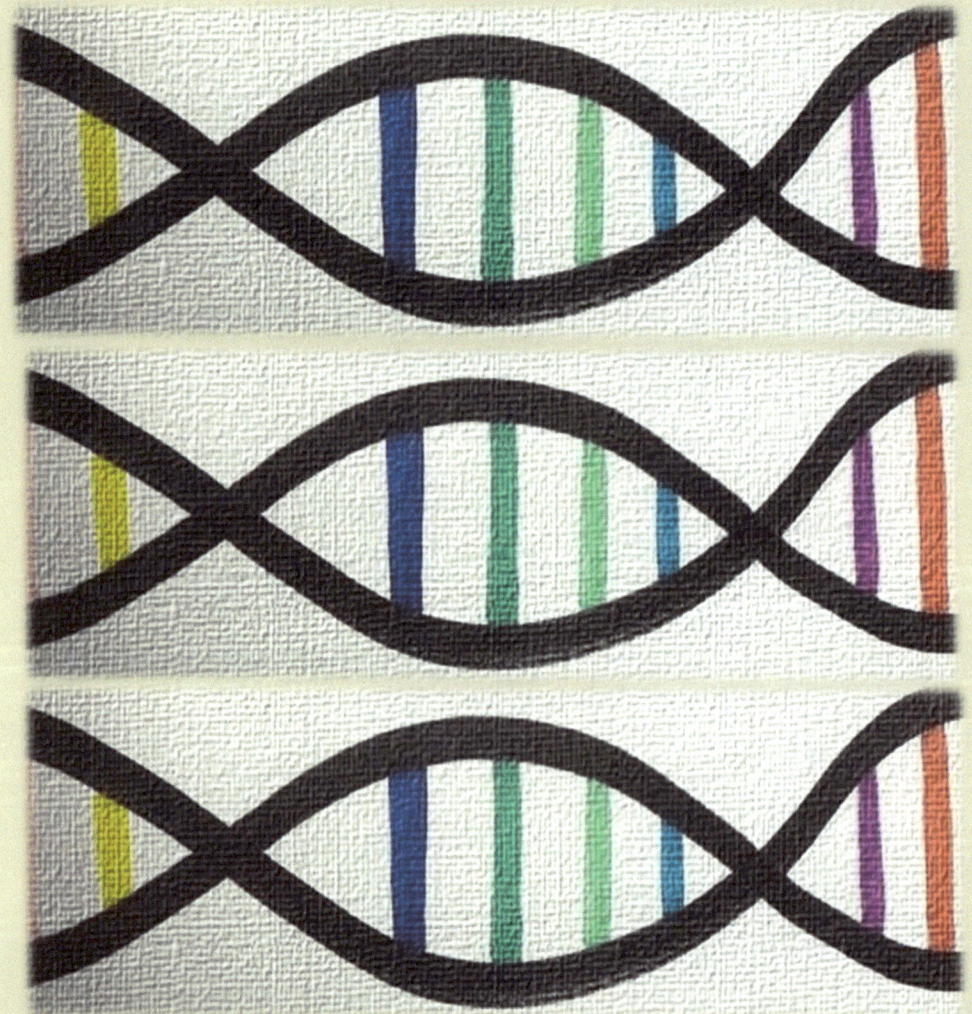

The cells in our bodies are always dying off, and we are constantly making new ones.

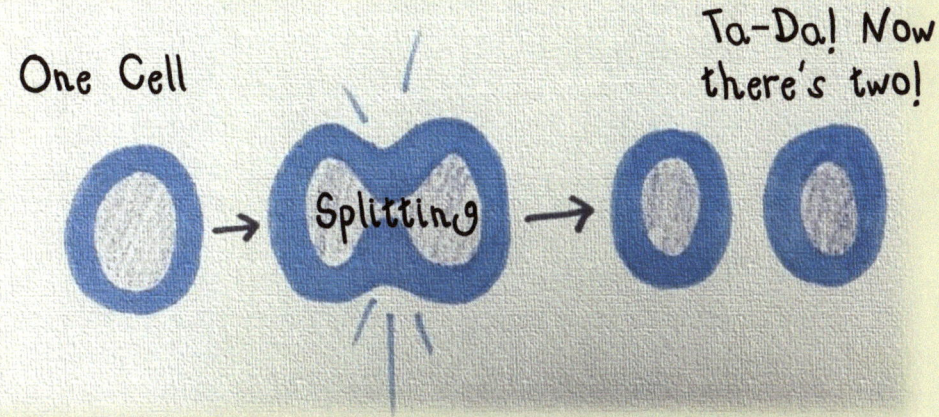

One Cell

→ Splitting →

Ta-Da! Now there's two!

In order for our bodies to make new cells, our DNA tells each cell to split apart and turn into two perfectly identical cells.

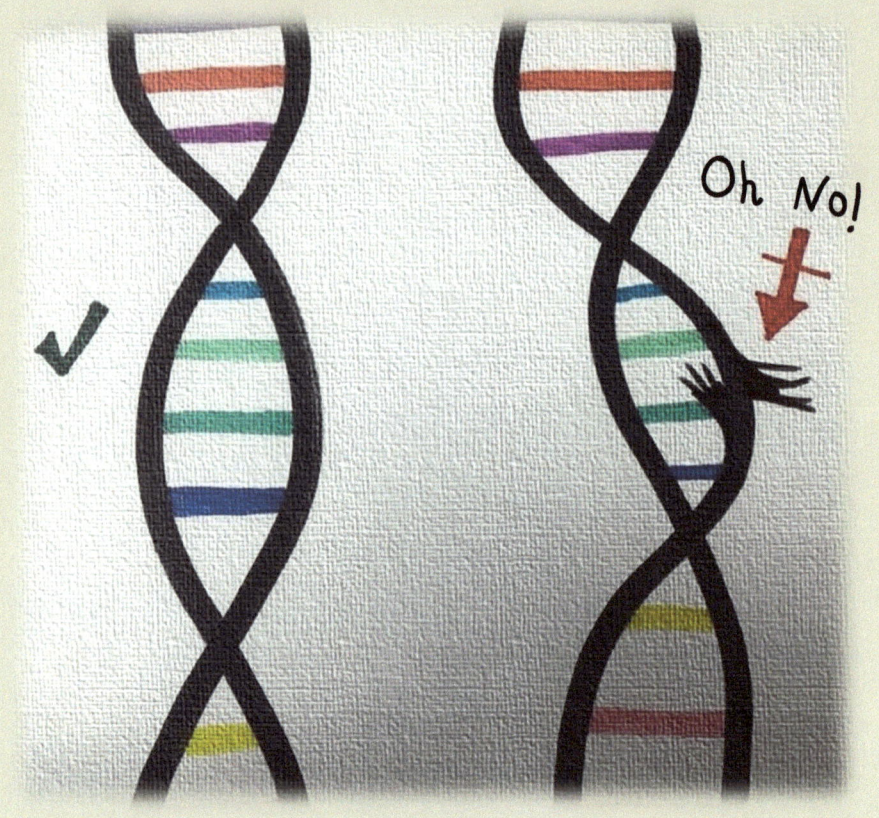

Sometimes the DNA gets damaged and isn't able to tell the cells what they need to do. This can cause the cells to get out of control!

When the body's cells are out of control, they act a little crazy. They keep splitting and growing at a very fast rate.

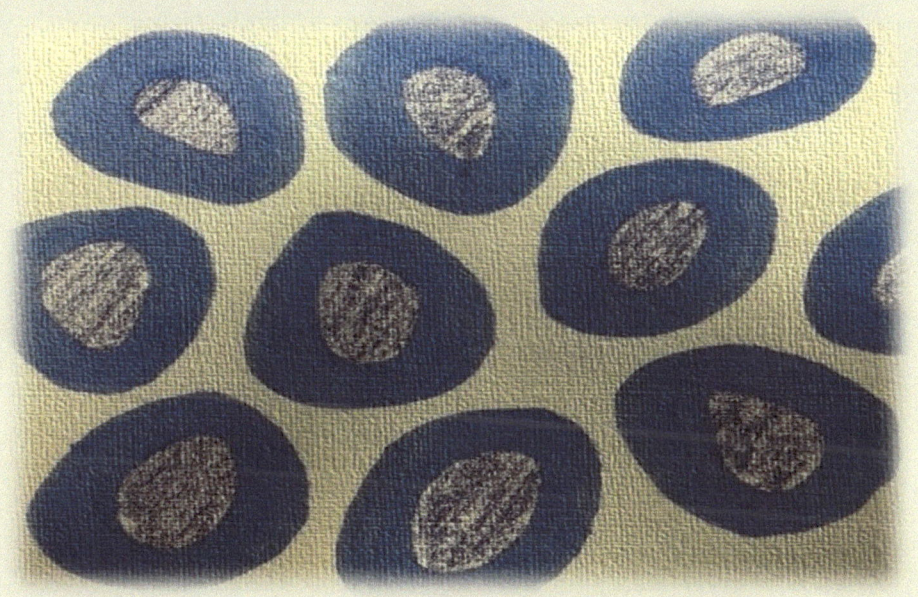

This causes the body to be jam-packed with new, healthy cells as well as old, sick ones.

Without the DNA to tell them what to do, the cells forget everything! They forget what they are, they forget what they do... they even forget to die!

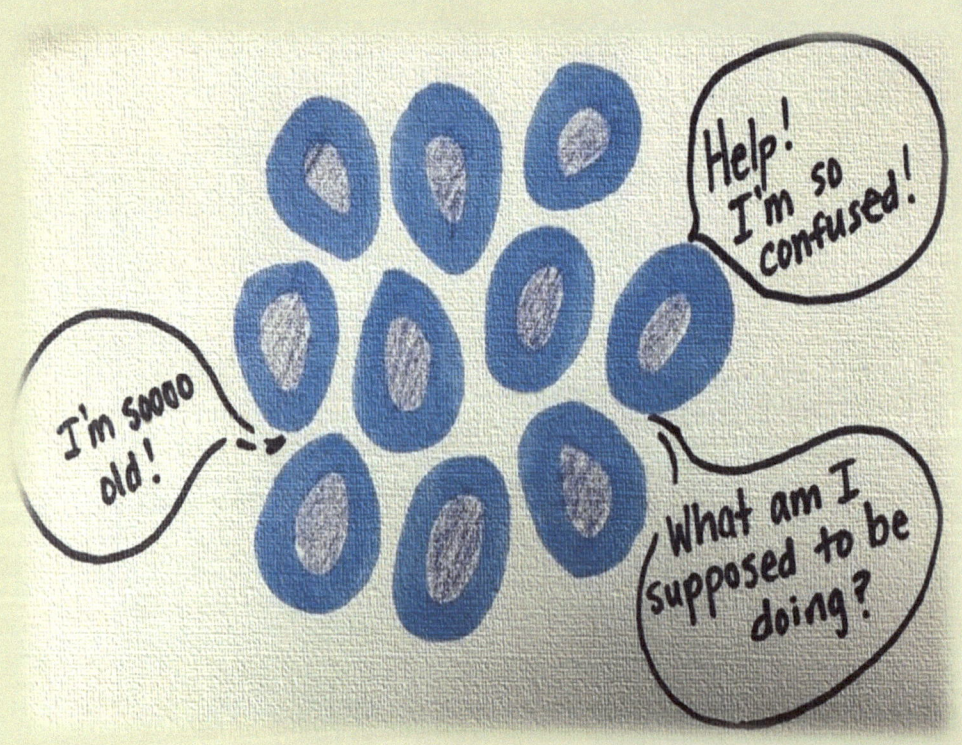

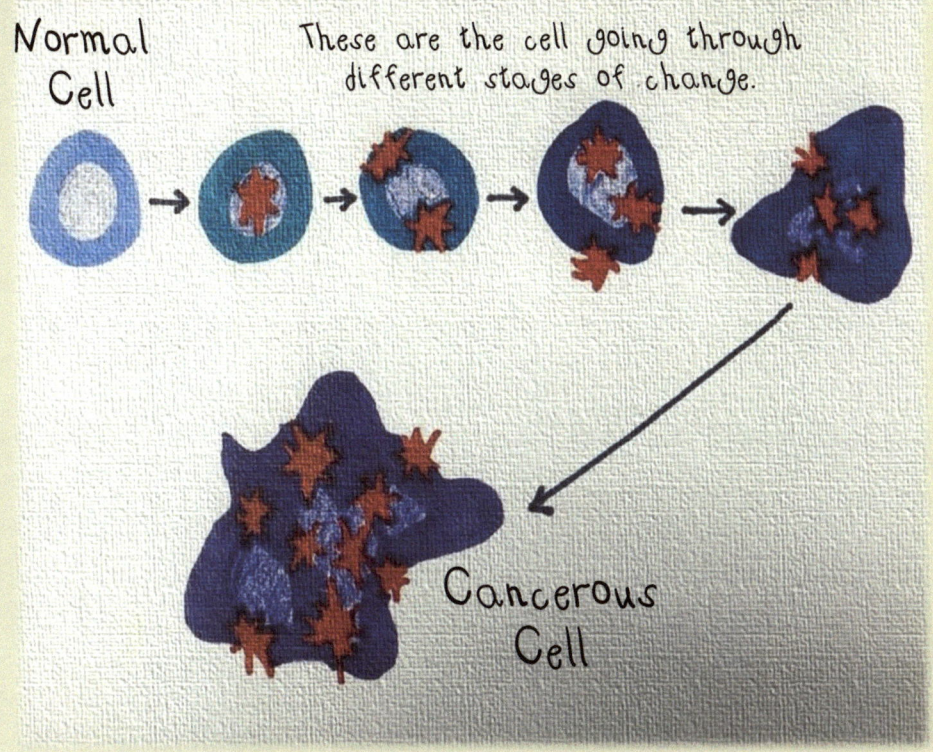

As these cells split and grow, they also change. This change and crowding of cells is called **cancer**.

Cancerous cells can live anywhere in the human body. Sometimes they are in a person's blood or bones, and other times the cells stick together and form a big clump. When that happens, it is called a tumor.

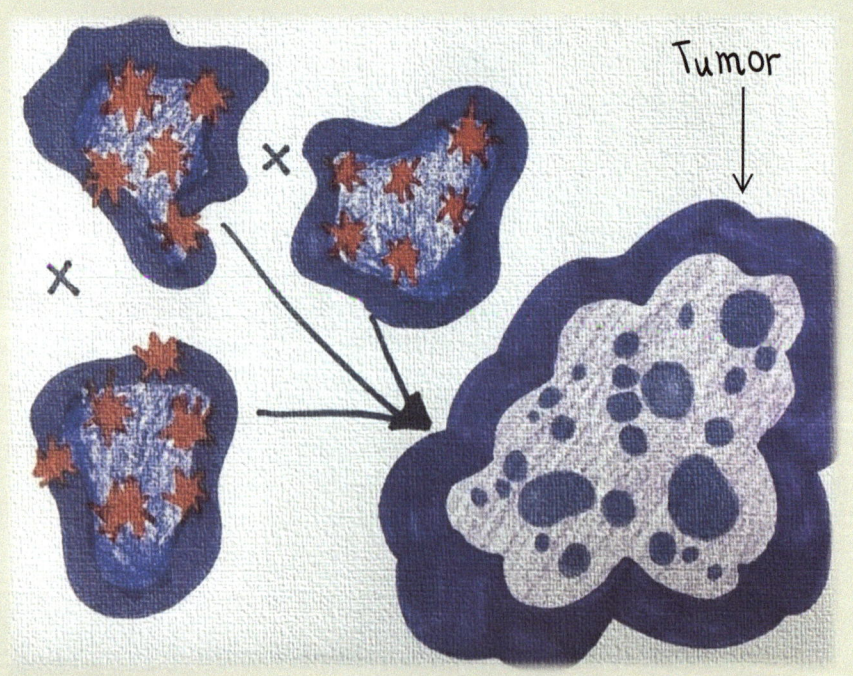

Tumor

There are many different types of cancer, but don't worry...cancer is **not** contagious!

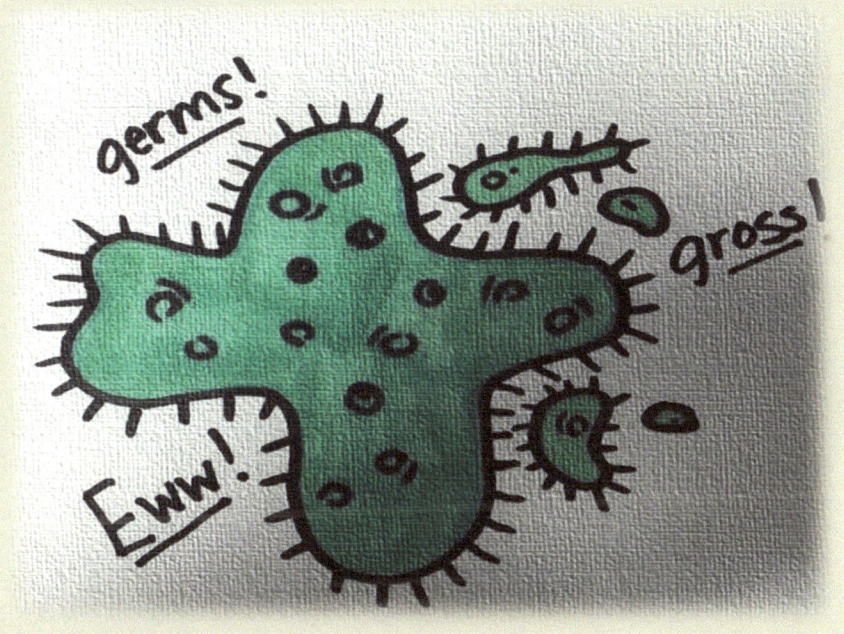

You can't catch cancer from anyone. It is not a germ and it can't be spread like the cold or flu.

BUT...

It is
important
to Know
that cancer
can happen
to anyone...
someone you
Know, and
even
someone you
love.

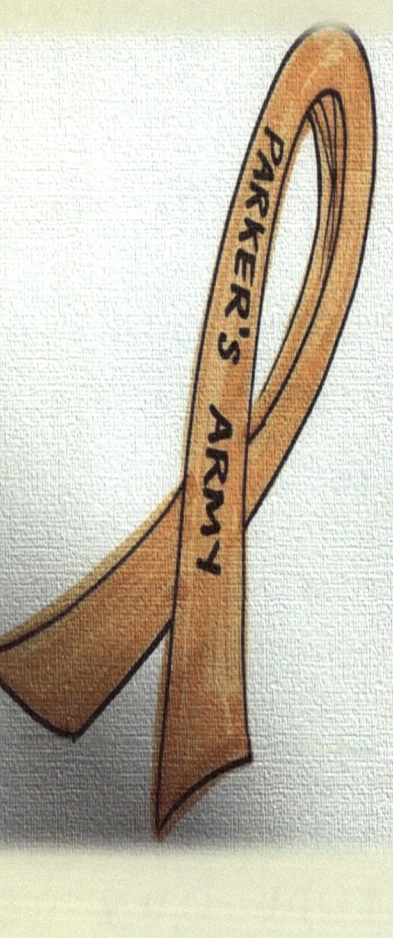

When a person learns that they have cancer they usually go to the hospital.

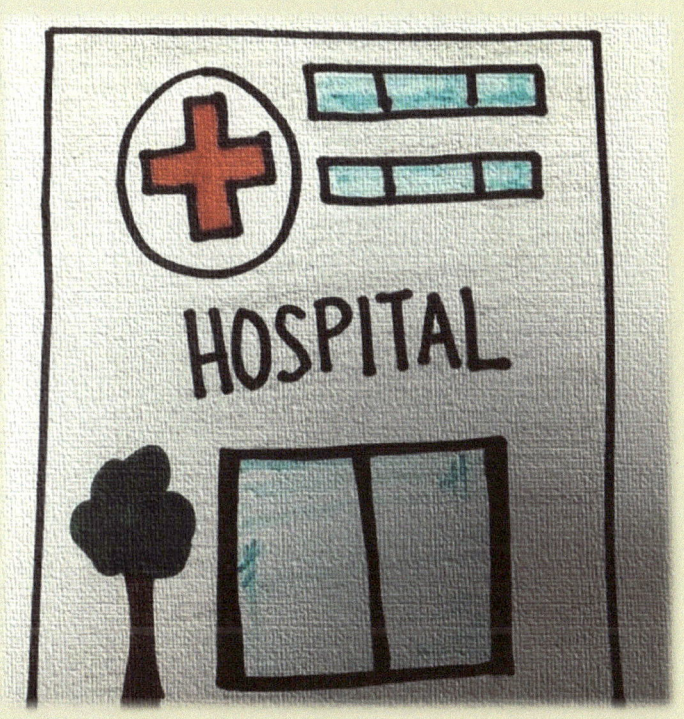

The doctors and nurses at the hospital will do lots of tests. These tests will help them decide what is the best way to get rid of the cancer.

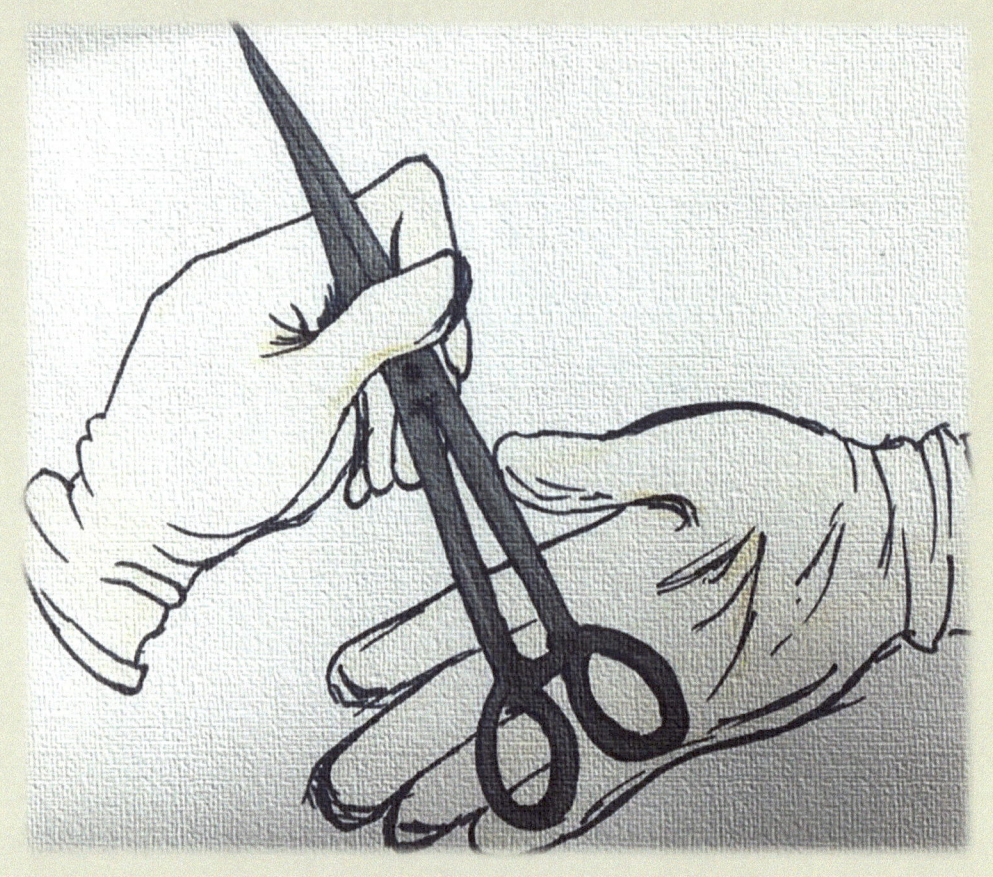

Sometimes the person will have surgery to remove the cancer from their body.

(This is the easiest way to get rid of most tumors.)

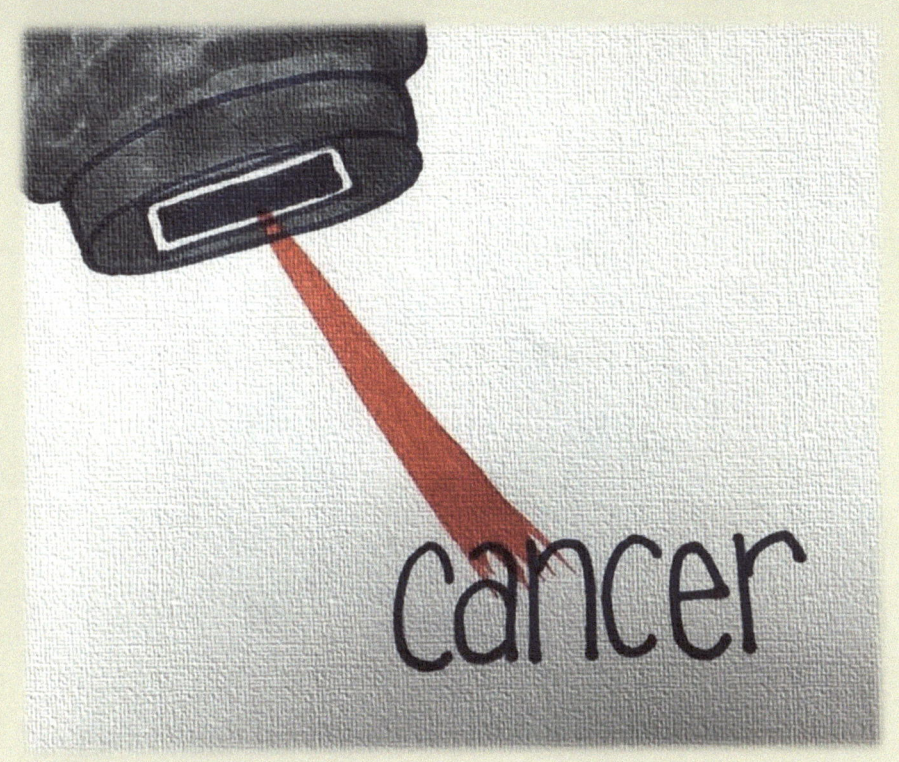

Other types of cancer can't be taken care of with surgery. Some of these cancers need radiation therapy.

This works by shooting beams of very intense energy directly at the cancer - which helps kill the cancer cells.

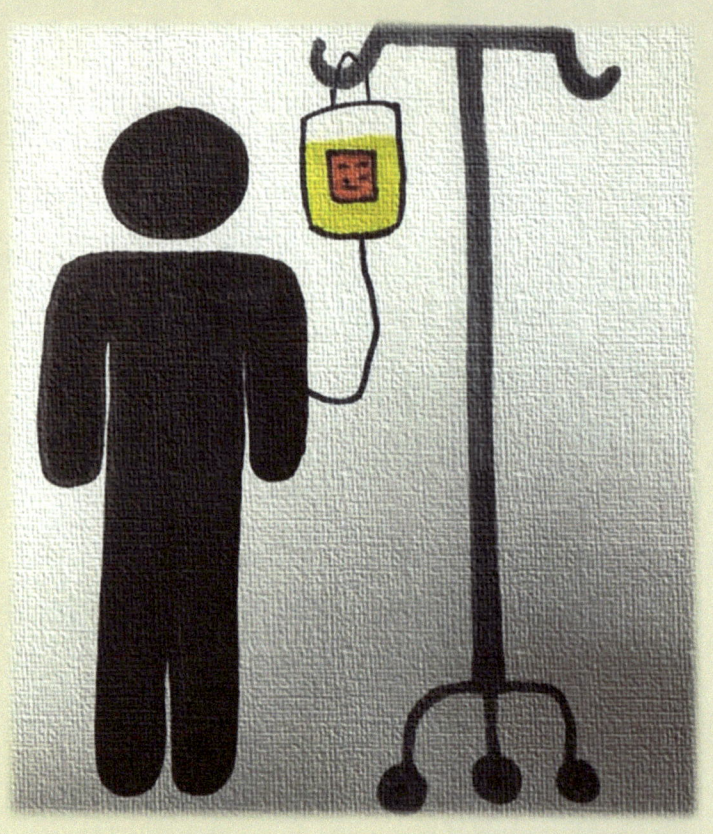

Many people also need
chemotherapy. (We call this
"chemo" for short.)

Chemo works by pumping
medicine into the person's body.
When it is in the body it can
run through their blood and
destroy the cells!

While these treatments are needed to get rid of the cancer cells, they sadly get rid of the GOOD cells in a person's body too.

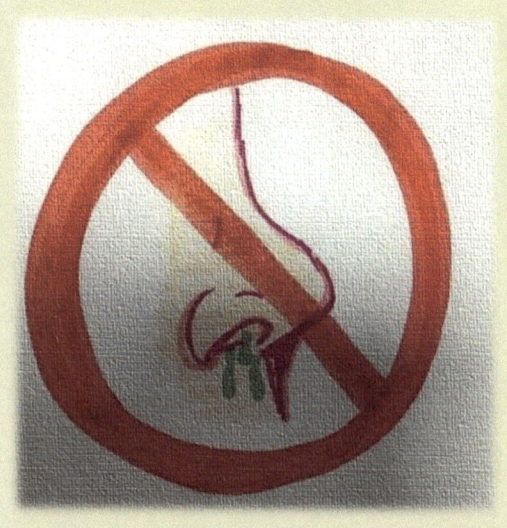

Without the good cells to protect their body from other germs, we must be very careful around people with cancer. We can easily spread our germs to them — without even knowing it!

Here are a few rules to follow if you know somebody with cancer:

✓ Stay away from them if you feel sick at all. Even if you have a little cough!

✓ Wash your hands before getting close to them.

✓ You may hug them, but your mouth carries too many germs to kiss them.

✓ Remember that they get tired easily, so let them have their rest.

✓ Don't forget that they are still a person. When someone has cancer, it is just a disease they are fighting, not who they really are!

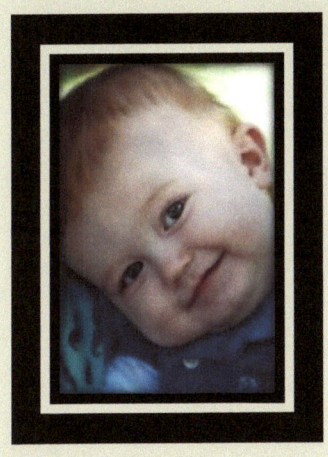

Parker's Story: Acute Myeloid Leukemia (AML)

Written in collaboration with Heather Norris
September 2, 2016

Parker has always been a happy little boy; active, chunky, and full of spunk. Although seemingly healthy, Parker quite frequently battled respiratory and ear infections; which ultimately led to him receiving ear tubes before his first birthday.

This summer was a tough one for Parker and his family, they couldn't seem to beat this latest round of ear infections. After many emergency room and doctor visits, being on multiple trials of antibiotics, Parker continued to have increased drainage out of his ears; along with continuous and high fevers. Doctors were stumped at the time, and so were Parker's parents, Kiefer and Jordan Hopkins. Parker is their second child, and they've dealt with these types of things before.

However, after another emergency room trip, it was soon realized that Parker was a very sick little boy. Lab test were drawn and revealed an extremely elevated white blood cell count, as well as very low platelet and hemoglobin levels; most often a tell-tale sign of Leukemia.

Parker's journey with AML began on Saturday, August 13, 2016; just two months shy of his second birthday.

At first, doctors suspected that Parker had Acute Lymphocytic Leukemia (ALL) and gave Kiefer and Jordan the statistics and a projected treatment plan; the survival rate is 98 percent with a chemotherapy over a course of three and a half years. In the whirlwind of the devastating circumstances, this was a relief. This led them to embrace a positive mind-set. Things could be worse; ALL is very curable, and their family would not bow to this obstacle; it was merely a challenge that their son would conquer.

On Monday, (August 15, 2016) Parker underwent a bone marrow biopsy, lumbar puncture, and port placement. He had some complications during the procedures, which ultimately required him to be on a ventilator overnight in the Pediatric Intensive Care Unit (PICU). After the test results came back, it was ultimately revealed that Parker did not have ALL.

Parker's diagnosis was less favorable than originally suspected; he had Acute Myeloid Leukemia, AML. Not only was the leukemia present in his blood, it was also detected in his cerebrospinal fluid; which is the fluid that surrounds the brain and spinal cord.

The switch of the diagnoses changed the course of Parker's treatment to four rounds of intense chemotherapy. Each round will last between four and six weeks, coinciding with semi-weekly lumbar punctures; directly injecting chemotherapy into the cerebrospinal fluid. The lumbar punctures will continue twice a week, every week, until the CSF is tested and comes back three times with no traces of leukemia present.

Parker is tolerating his first 28 day round of chemo surprisingly well, although he will likely spend his second birthday as an inpatient at the University of Iowa Children's Hospital. Like all toddlers, Parker has his good days and his bad days. However, his bad days aren't caused by the simple things most his age experience.

When Parker is unsettled, crying, or throwing a fit, it isn't because he missed his afternoon nap or because he didn't get the biggest cookie on the plate; he is disheartened because he is suffering.

He is mentally and physically exhausted. Parker is tired; every inch of his body, inside and out, hurts.

If the chemotherapy does not work for Parker, the next option is to have a bone marrow transplant. This is why Parker's family and friends are strongly encouraging people to go to https://join.bethematch.org/Parker and register to be a bone marrow donor.

When individuals are conquering battles such as Parker's, people often say "Nobody Fights Alone," and that has proven to be very true for this little boy and his family. In just 24 hours, the Muscatine community, Parker's family, and friends rallied together to raise more than $3,000 in a GoFundMe account. And as of today, the monetary donation balance is just under $11,000!

Individuals and businesses; both near and far, have generously donated items to raffle at a benefit planned for October 1st, 2016. Several local bars and eateries have hosted benefit nights, where they donated a percent of their sales to #ParkerStrong and #ParkersArmy. These are merely a few of the great things happening in the Muscatine community to support Parker, and there are many more benefits, yard sales and raffles to come.

#ParkerStrong and #ParkersArmy are trending on social media, and can be seen just about anywhere you look on the internet. #ParkerStrong is a brand that started to highlight Parker's story, so family members, friends, and all of his supporters could stay updated on his progress. #ParkersArmy is another brand that was started, for not only Parker, but for everyone fighting some type of war; because whether we realize it or not, we are all battling something.

For Parker's mother, Jordan, second to Parker's leukemia, her own education is the battle. Jordan is in her first year of nursing school, and despite discouragement to continue in the nursing program, Jordan is determined to continue with classes while Parker is receiving treatment at the University of Iowa Hospital.

Her husband, Kiefer, is what most would consider the Platoon Leader for his soldiers. Since Parker's diagnosis, Kiefer has been unable to work due to his family's needs. He has been committed to ensuring that Parker's three-year-old brother, Maddux is happy, loved, and cared for, is Parker's battle buddy during this war, and is making it possible for his wife to continue her education, so that she may be victorious for her troops.

Just a few days into this crusade, Parker's uncle Justin gave his family, as well as all of #ParkersArmy, knowledgeable and encouraging words. He said "As long as we progress 1% each day, we are winning our battle. If we can do something 1% better each day, we are never going backwards."

Although it has been about three weeks since his diagnosis, the reality of things are starting to really set in — as Parker's hair begins to fall out, and his skin pales, he hasn't lost his sense of humor. He fights everyday with a smile on his face, and generally an Oreo (or five) in his hands, showing what #ParkerStrong really means.